I0424892

The Healthy Pregnancy Plan

Written by
Martha Diebold

"Feeling fat lasts nine months but the joy of becoming a mom lasts forever."

- Nikki Dalton

Contents

Introduction

If you suspect, or know, that you are pregnant, we hope you have already visited your doctor!

Presuming that you have confirmed your suspicions and that this is your first child, or that you wish to take better care of yourself during pregnancy than you did during your other pregnancies; you have come to the right place!

My goal is to give pregnant women over the age of 30 all the information they will need to care for their health and the health of their unborn child during their pregnancy.

To do that, I believe it is important for you to understand pregnancy, and what is happening to your body as your baby develops and nears term.

Therefore, all the information I give you about taking care of yourself will be clarified with information about what is happening to your body and why it is important to follow the recommendations I give you and the recommendations and advice of your doctor.

First, and foremost, it is important to consult a doctor and to get on a schedule of visits and testing to accommodate every stage of your pregnancy.

If you are healthy and expect a normal pregnancy, you have some options for health care during your pregnancy:

➢ *Obstetrician/Gynecologist (OB/GYN)* – these doctors have a specialty in pregnancy and women's health.

➢ *Family General Practitioner or Internist* – doctors who provide standard medical care to all men and women and in some cases will provide obstetrical care.

Although, malpractice insurance for this type of medical care has sharply increased, so in many cases, general practitioners (GPS) and internists no longer delivery babies, or treat women during the pregnancy term.

So, many of these doctors will no longer care for a pregnant woman, but instead will refer you to an OB/GYN.

➢ *Nurse/Midwives* – these health care professionals specialize in women's health and follow a pregnant mother through prenatal care, and labor and delivery.

Nurse/Midwives need a doctor 'on call' for the delivery in case there is a problem during delivery.

They also provide post partum care for normal pregnancies, referring women to an OB/GYN for complications or specific health related issues. Be sure your midwife is certified, and fully trained!

When you visit your doctor for the first time, he/she will perform blood tests and a pelvic exam to confirm your pregnancy, *and estimate a due date.*

We'll talk a little about due dates later when we discuss the first trimester.

The blood test detects HCG (human chorionic gonadotropin). HCG is a hormone produced by a woman's body after an egg has been fertilized and a woman's pregnancy commences.

HCG can be detected in blood or urine even before a missed period, as early as six to eight days after conception.

HCG levels will significantly increase during the first trimester and then decrease a bit throughout the remainder of the pregnancy.

Abnormal HCG levels can indicate a possible miscarriage or a tubal pregnancy, or it may mean the mother can expect a multiple birth (twins, triplets, etc).

Your doctor will talk to you about any abnormality in your HCG levels and monitor these levels throughout your pregnancy.

Assuming your HCG levels are consistent with a normal pregnancy, this test will not be performed again.

Doctor visits and examinations should also into consideration your family history, and any pre-existing health problems you may have.

You should also tell your doctor about any special circumstances you may need to accommodate because of your job or your family situation.

During your pregnancy, your doctor may or will perform certain tests, depending on your individual situation. We have included a list of these tests here.

You will find a routine doctor's visit schedule included in the list below.

Remember that your individual situation may vary, but this list will give you an idea of when and how often you will need to see your doctor and what tests may be performed while you are there.

First exam and HCG test	6 to 8 weeks into your term
Chorionic villus sampling (CVS)	10 to 12 weeks into your term
Second doctor's visit	10 to 12 weeks into your term
Amniocentesis	15 to 18 weeks into your term
Third doctor's visit	14 to 16 weeks into your term
Multiple marker screening	15 to 20 weeks into your term
Fourth doctor's visit	18 to 20 weeks in your term
Ultrasound	16 to 20 weeks into your term
Fifth doctor's visit	22 to 24 weeks into your term
Glucose screening test (GCT)	24 to 28 weeks into your term
Sixth doctor's visit	26 to 28 weeks into your term
Doctor's visit	Every two weeks from 28th to 36th week
Group B strep screening	35 to 37 weeks into your term
Doctor's visit	Once a week 37th week through delivery

When you go to the doctor, she will check your weight, your blood pressure and your abdomen, check your baby's heart beat, and usually do a pelvic exam.

Some women are uncomfortable with these types of intimate exams and they do take some getting used to, if you are not accustomed to annual OB/GYN exams and pap smears.

But, these exams ARE very important to your health and to the health of your baby.

So, stick with it.

Don't miss appointments, and don't assume everything is OK because you don't feel you have any symptoms or problems. Let your health care professional do her/his job!

Remember that once you know you are pregnant, it is very important to take care of yourself.

You will get lots of advice from everyone – even strangers – about what you should do and what you should NOT do.

It is important to be educated and informed, especially if this is your first baby, so that you feel confident that you know what you are doing.

Otherwise, you are likely to be blown in the wind as people give conflicting advice, and you will feel scattered and uncertain.

Before we dive into the details of this book, we thought you might like to make note of this website link.

As you talk to your healthcare professional, you are likely to hear some words you have not heard before.
Of course, you should always ask your doctor to explain what you don't understand.

But, if you want to do some research on your own, or if you hear a word you want to research in between visits, you can use this handy guide to commonly used pregnancy terms:

Glossary

http://www.happyhealthypregnancy.com/info/pregnancy_tools/preg_terms.aspx

Now, let's move on.

Chapter 1: Symptoms and Considerations During Pregnancy

In this section of the book, we will talk about general concerns and describe some of the issues, symptoms and feelings you may have during pregnancy.

These are general descriptions, meant to give you an idea of what is normal and when you should be concerned.

As always, if you have a question or become concerned, you should contact your doctor.

In the sections that follow you will find guidelines for nutrition and exercise, and a lot of helpful information on the changes that occur during each trimester.

And you'll find out how to take care of your body and adjust your schedule and your life style during each stage of your pregnancy.

After you find out you are pregnant, after the excitement and buzz has worn off, you should expect the physical reality to set in.

During pregnancy you may experience fatigue, tenderness in your breasts, morning sickness, etc. Not every woman has every symptom.

Some women SAIL through pregnancy and others seem to endure lots of little problems that don't amount of anything serious, but are enough to disrupt life in general.

Here are some of the things you may encounter during pregnancy:

Fatigue – You may feel 'bone tired' or become easily fatigued during pregnancy, especially in your first trimester.

Remember that your body is working harder producing certain hormones and supplying blood and nutrients to your baby in the womb.

One of the hormones, progesterone, is a central nervous system depressant, so this hormone can make you feel drowsy or sleepy.

Try to pamper yourself during this time. Many women find that after their first trimester, they have renewed energy and stamina. In the meantime, take naps or just rest if you can.

Bleeding – It is not unusual to have a small amount of spotting or bleeding early in pregnancy – around 10 to 14 days after conception.

This bleeding is a bit earlier, spottier and 'pinker' in color than a usual menstrual cycle and it doesn't last very long.

Talk to your doctor and let him know about this, but don't be concerned unless the bleeding is heavy and lasts a long time. You may also get a bit of cramping early in pregnancy.

Changes in Appetite or Food Preferences - The smell of some foods may cause nausea during early pregnancy.

Or you may find you have a craving for certain foods during late pregnancy. The famous 'ice cream and pickles' legend is not so far from the truth for some women!

Many women find that they can no longer abide coffee during early pregnancy, and that this aversion subsides as their pregnancy progresses.

Among the foods that may wreak havoc on your stomach: Meat, cheese or milk, and spicy foods. Don't be surprised if these preferences and aversions change as your pregnancy progresses.

Morning Sickness, Nausea and Vomiting - Typically confined to early pregnancy, though some women experience this symptom for up to six months.

Most women encounter morning sickness for about a month during their first trimester, and symptoms can start as early as 14 days after conception.

Morning sickness is not always confined to the morning, and it results from the changing levels of estrogen in the body.

Some women experience morning sickness with no trigger, while others will become nauseous from certain smells like cigarette or cigar smoke, strong perfume, coffee or the smell of certain foods cooking.

Increased Urination – As your uterus enlarges, you are likely to feel the urge to go to the bathroom more often. This is normal during the first and third trimester.

Breast Tenderness and Changes - Increased production of the estrogen and progesterone is required to prepare the breasts for nursing.

During the early stages of pregnancy, some women complain that their breasts become so tender and sensitive that they can't even sleep on their stomach or touch the tissue on their breasts without discomfort.

This tenderness does pass. Women who are flat-chested often welcome the changes that pregnancy brings, as their breasts increase in size.

Be sure to buy and wear a comfortable bra, with plenty of support, during and after pregnancy to accommodate these changes. If you are planning to nurse your baby, you will want to look for special 'nursing bras' to make nursing easier.

Headaches - Many pregnant women complain of mild headaches that occur frequently, early in pregnancy. These headaches occur because of increased blood circulation caused by hormonal fluctuation and changes in the body.

Constipation and Bloating – Constipation is common during early pregnancy because of an increase in progesterone that slows digestion. Drink plenty of water to keep your body hydrated and help ease constipation and bloating.

Mood Fluctuation – Again, it is all due to the hormonal changes in your body. You may be an even-tempered person and suddenly find yourself crying or losing your temper for no reason.

Understand that these mood swings are common during the first trimester and will usually improve.

Dizziness - Early in your pregnancy you may feel dizzy or faint because of low blood sugar and changes in circulation and hormone levels.

Be sure to drink plenty of water and keep crackers and other healthy snacks on hand to address low blood sugar and don't be surprised if you need to rest and pamper yourself a bit more, especially during early pregnancy.

Weight Gain and Changes in Center of Gravity – Your balance and center of gravity are going to change as your body changes.

Don't try to walk a tightrope or a ladder in your new, 'enhanced' condition!

Wear sensible shoes without high heels so you can balance and walk more easily without falling or stumbling.

Most mothers gain 25 to 35 pounds, some as much as 50-60 pounds during pregnancy.
And that additional can make you uncomfortable, causing back strain and soreness. 50% of all pregnant women develop low-back pain at some time during their pregnancy.

Be sure to use your legs when you are lifting and use common sense when lifting or climbing during pregnancy.

Increased and displaced weight puts more stress on joints and as the baby grows, your lower back must compensate for this weight.

We'll talk about exercise in a little while, but for now, understand that it is important to keep your muscles strong and limber during this time, in order to avoid back strain and fatigue.

Chapter 2: Guidelines for Good Health

Nutrition

Now that you are pregnant, it is no time to diet. You certainly want to eat the right things and try not to gain an unhealthy amount of weight, but you should NOT be dieting right now.

> ➤ You will need about 300 to 350 calories more per day than when you were eating just for you – about 2,500 to 2,700 calories per day.

> ➤ If you are very thin by nature or if you are going through a multiple birth pregnancy, your doctor may even prescribe more of an increase in daily caloric intake.

> ➤ On the other hand, if you are typically overweight, your doctor may advise that you consume more calories, but she may advise you to drop below the additional 300 to 350 usually prescribed for an average pregnancy.

You should plan to maintain a well-balanced diet throughout your pregnancy, consisting of lean meats and protein, fruits, vegetables, and *whole-grain* breads, as well as *low-fat* dairy products like cheese and milk.

Your doctor will probably prescribe prenatal vitamins for you. These are special vitamins compounded with the correct amounts of calcium, iron and folic acid needed by pregnant women.

Don't make the mistake of thinking that your prenatal vitamins will cover all the nutritional needs you have.

You still need to eat well!

We have provided details here, so that you can build a good nutritional base for your own health, and for the health of your unborn child. *As always, if you have any questions throughout the course of your pregnancy,, please consult your doctor.*

Let's look at the details of your nutritional building blocks:

Vegetables and Fruits – 4 or more servings of vegetables and 3 or more servings of fruits, at minimum.

Here are some examples of serving sizes:

Fruits: One medium-sized apple or banana, one half cup of chopped fruit or three quarters of a cup of fruit juice.

Vegetables: One cup of leafy vegetable (raw), one half cup of non-leafy vegetable (either cooked or raw) or three quarters of a cup of a vegetable juice (like tomato juice)

Eating fruits and vegetables that contain Vitamin C will help you absorb iron, heal minor wounds and maintain healthy gums and body tissue. Examples of these types of vegetables and fruits include:

Fruits: Papaya, tomato, orange, melon, strawberry

Vegetables: Peppers, cabbage, broccoli, green leafy vegetables like spinach and escarole.

Protein - Two or more servings of lean, cooked meat or poultry (without the skin), or fish. These servings should amount to 60 grams of protein per day.

Here are some examples of serving sizes:

Meat, Poultry, Fish: Two to three ounces of cooked meat, poultry or fish. Do NOT eat *undercooked* or *UNCOOKED* meat, poultry or fish. These may contain bacteria and can make you very sick! Avoid 'lunch meat', 'cold cuts' or 'deli meats'.

Try to stay away from fish with high mercury content (shark, swordfish, tilefish (white snapper or golden snapper) and king mackerel.

These fish tend to contain more mercury content, which can be harmful to your baby. Do not eat more than six ounces of tuna or tuna steak per week.

If you need more information on mercury levels in fish, use this website:
http://www.cfsan.fda.gov/~frf/sea-mehg.html

Other Proteins: One third cup of nuts, 1
                                   cooked egg, one half cup of
                                   tofu or cooked beans or
                                   peas, or two tablespoons of
                                   peanut butter.

Eating protein helps you to build muscle, and keeps you healthy and strong. It also helps your body to provide antibodies for your baby. Protein contains the B Vitamins and iron important to produce rich, red blood cells and keep your blood strong.

Protein is especially important during your second and third trimester, as it will help your body keep up with the demands and growth of your baby in the womb.

Whole Grains and Whole Grain Products - Nine or more servings of whole grain products per day. *Try to stay away from white flour, sweetened cereals, etc.* They contain little or no nutritional value.

Here are some examples of serving sizes:

Whole Wheat or Other Whole Grain Bread:

One slice

Cooked (hot) Cereal, Brown Rice or Whole Grain Pasta:

One half cup

Cold Cereal:

One cup

These products contain B Vitamins, and minerals and fiber to keep your body healthy and keep your digestive system moving.

Folic acid is often added to cold breakfast cereals and to 'enriched' grain products and this is also an important mineral for your body during pregnancy. Look at the packaging and try to choose products that contain more folic acid, wherever possible.

Dairy Products - Four or more servings per day. While you are pregnant, you will want to consume about at least 1,000 mg (milligrams) of calcium per day (1,300 milligrams if you are under eighteen years of age).

If you cannot get that much calcium in your diet, ask your doctor about your prenatal vitamins to be sure that you are getting enough calcium by looking at your combined diet and supplements.

If you find that you are lactose intolerant, you can use reduced lactose products, or take tablets to increase your tolerance of dairy products. Talk to your doctor to find out which solution will work best for you.

Here are some examples of serving sizes of dairy products:

Cheese (natural, not processed): One and one half ounces

Low-Fat or Non-Fat Milk: One cup

Natural (active ingredient) Yogurt: One cup

You and your growing baby both need lots of calcium to keep your bones and your teeth strong. Dairy products contain Vitamins A and D, and also protein, and B Vitamins. Vitamin A is important for your baby's growth, and for immune system support.

Water – 6-8 eight ounce glasses of water per day (if you are exercising: 8-10 glasses)

This may seem like a lot but your body will adjust to this volume, and you need to stay hydrated during pregnancy to prevent constipation, hemorrhoids, swelling, dehydration, urinary and bladder infections, and muscle strain.

Vitamins and Minerals

We've talked about how important it is to follow a good diet during pregnancy. Your prenatal vitamins, combined with the good food you eat should give you enough of the right vitamins and minerals.

If you look at the label of your prenatal vitamin bottle, you should see plenty of the following vitamins and minerals.

Calcium - Most women don't get enough calcium (1,000 mg per day) but when you are pregnant your need for calcium is even more important, to meet the demands of your body and the demands of your baby's calcium needs to grow strong bones.

Be sure your prenatal vitamins contain 1,000 mg (1,300 if you are under eighteen) per dose.

Iron – You need iron to produce hemoglobin and red blood cells. Hemoglobin is the component of red blood cells that carries oxygen throughout your system.

It supplies all your cells and your baby's body and organs with plenty of rich oxygenated blood with which to grow and remain healthy.

Your body and your baby's body also need iron to grow bones and teeth and to prevent anemia. Be sure your prenatal vitamins contain 27 to 30 mg of iron per dose.

Folic Acid (Folate) - Studies show that taking folic acid supplements during pregnancy decreases the risk of neural tube defects by up to 70%!

The neural tube contains your baby's spinal cord and developing brain, and when it does not form properly it can cause serious conditions like spina bifida, and congenital heart disease.

Because your body uses folic acid very early in pregnancy, it is wise to start taking a supplement if you are planning a pregnancy.

Check your prenatal vitamins to be sure you are getting 400 micrograms (0.4 milligrams) per dose.

Chapter 3: Pregnancy and Diabetes

If you are a diabetic and you want to get pregnant, work with your OB/GYN doctor and your diabetes doctor to be sure you are in the best shape possible *at least three to six months* before you conceive.

Then be sure you are followed regularly by both physicians so that you remain healthy during your pregnancy and after delivery.

During your pregnancy you should monitor your diet and exercise program and look for signs of imbalance in your blood sugar, as pregnancy can sometimes wreak havoc on your regular routine and your insulin levels.

You may have to get a special meal plan from a nutritionist or dietician in order to compensate for the changes in your body and your blood sugar and ensure that your child does not experience problems or birth defects because of high blood sugar levels that may cross into the placenta.

Talk to your doctor about getting more B Vitamins, especially folic acid to guard against the risk of birth defects.

If you have never been diabetic in the past, you may find yourself facing 'gestational diabetes', which is a form of diabetes that occurs during pregnancy and typically disappears after delivery.

This form of diabetes is usually controlled with diet, medication, and exercise, but it must be treated in order to ensure that you and your baby remain healthy.

Your OB/GYN doctor will usually refer you to a dietitian so you can get meal plans that are specially designed to help you control your blood sugar.

Chapter 4: Vegetarian Diets

If you are a strict 'vegan' and eat no animal products or animal byproducts, you may feel you will have a problem during pregnancy. Or perhaps you are a 'lacto-ovo-vegan' and you do eat eggs and dairy products.

If you wish to maintain a vegan diet during pregnancy, by all means you should find a doctor who is willing to support this approach and stay in close contact with her regarding your nutritional health and your baby's health, as your pregnancy progresses.

Here are some nutritional guidelines that will help you stay healthy and deliver a healthy baby.

To get all the protein and calcium you need – the biggest problem faced by most vegans – you will want to eat appropriate amounts of the following things:

- o dried peas (split peas are great),
- o dried beans (cooked) including navy beans, kidney or red beans, black or lima beans and white beans,

- soy products like tempeh, tofu and tofu cheese,
- almonds and other nuts, and butter made from nut oils,
- soy milk or goat milk or cow milk (if you drink it), and/or
- active yogurt
- turnip greens,
- oranges,
- broccoli,
- molasses,
- fortified cereals,
- wheat germ,
- spinach,
- raisins

The great thing about a vegetarian diet is that it is already high in folic acid and B Vitamins and that is important to your baby's health and growth.

However, you may find it hard to get your extra 300-350 calories per day if you are eating a vegetarian diet.

Your diet, while high in fiber, with plenty of vegetables, fruits and grains, tends to be low in calories and you don't feel hungry enough to eat more because all that fiber will fill you up!

Talk to your doctor about this, if you find that it is a problem. You may want to take a caloric supplement.

Chapter 5: Things You Should Avoid in Your Diet

What you DON'T eat or drink during your pregnancy can be just as important as what you DO consume!

Here are some things to avoid while you are pregnant:

Alcohol – We shouldn't have to tell you this, but we will anyway! STAY AWAY FROM ALCOHOL DURING PREGNANCY.

A glass of wine or bottle of beer may seem harmless enough but no study has yet to determine how much is a safe amount of alcohol and how much can cause mental retardation, central nervous system damage, brain damage, and birth defects in your baby.

It is better to be safe than sorry!
Alcohol goes straight into your baby's body in high concentration levels through your blood stream, through the umbilical cord and into the placenta, and can cause any one of an array of symptoms included in Fetal Alcohol Spectrum Disorder (FASD).

Children with FASD can have learning disabilities, memory and attention disorders, as well as language, and vision, or hearing problems, to name a few. So save that glass of wine or bottle of beer and enjoy it after you delivery your healthy child!

Caffeine – Consuming a lot of caffeine can increase your chance of miscarriage. Two or three cups a day may not seem like much to you, but just to be safe, you should try to stop drinking coffee altogether.

If you find you cannot do so, at least try to cut it down to one cup per day or start drinking decaffeinated coffee!

And remember that there are other beverages and foods that contain high concentrations of caffeine. Green tea and black tea, cola sodas (pop), even chocolate.

You can have these things in moderation (one cup of tea or a half of glass of soda or a candy bar once a week), because the caffeine content in these products is typically much less than that contained in cup of coffee (90-140 mg of caffeine).

You'll be happy to know that the average candy bar only contains 5-30 mg of caffeine, but you still need to consider the FAT content in that candy and remember the word:

MODERATION

Foods to Avoid

Avoid foods that MAY carry bacteria and other food-borne illness (toxoplasmosis and listeriosis to name two). These can cause birth defects and miscarriage, and while you may be able to eat them with no problems, you may not want to take the risk during your pregnancy.

- o Un-pasteurized (soft) cheeses, often labeled as 'fresh cheese' like feta cheese, goat cheese, brie, camembert, and blue or limburger cheeses.

- o Un-pasteurized milk, juice, or apple cider

- o Raw eggs or foods that contain raw eggs like tiramisu, mousse, cookie or cake batter, homemade ice cream, Caesar dressing (if made fresh).

- o Raw fish like sushi and CERTAINLY raw meat

○ High mercury content fish like shark, swordfish, tilefish (white snapper or golden snapper), and king mackerel

If you are a health advocate and you routinely take herbs, *please do NOT take* these particular herbs while you are pregnant:

Arbor Vitae	Autumn Crocus
Barberry	Basil Oil
Beth Root	Black Cohosh
Bloodroot	Blue Cohosh
Broom	Bugleweed
Clove Oil	Comfrey
Cotton Root	Devil's Claw
Dong Quai	False Unicorn Root
Feverfew	Golden Seal
Greater Celandine	Juniper and Juniper Oil
Lady's Mantle	Liferoot
Mistletoe	Mugwort (avoid during pregnancy & breast feeding)

American Pennyroyal European Pennyroyal (avoid during pregnancy & breast feeding)

Peruvian Bark   Pokeroot

Pseudoginseng Pulsatilla (limit use while breast feeding)

Rue   Sassafras

Shepherd's Purse   Southernwood (avoid during
pregnancy & breast feeding)

Squill   Tansy

Wild yam   Wormwood (avoid during
pregnancy & breast feeding)

Chapter 6: Exercise

Unless you have a serious problem or abnormality in your pregnancy, you should expect to continue to exercise throughout your term.

If you have NOT exercised in the past, you will, of course, want to consult your doctor to determine the level and frequency of exercise you can do during your pregnancy.

Exercise during pregnancy is healthy and will help to reduce swelling and bloat, prevent excessive weight gain, reduce muscle and back strain, and constipation, improve your energy levels, your sleep patterns and your mood.

It will also help you stay in shape for labor and reduce your recovery time after delivery.

The best kind of exercise during pregnancy is exercise with moderate strain and intensity (brisk walking, and swimming are great choices).

There are also yoga and Pilates classes designed specifically for pregnant women to provide them with strength conditioning, and flexibility.

Many of these classes are available on video and DVD so look in your local book store or online.

Meditation and relaxation classes are also great to relieve work, family and pregnancy related stress and to prepare you mentally and emotionally for the delivery marathon.

Remaining calm and relaxed can ease your delivery tremendously and these techniques should not be overlooked.

Remember that it is just as important to exercise and prepare your brain as it is to exercise your body!

Avoid exercise like high-impact aerobics, rock climbing, gymnastics that require balance or exercise at high elevations. Don't water ski, snow ski or ride a horse and use common sense when exercising during pregnancy.

Always ask your doctor before undertaking or pursuing an exercise program.

You should also know that among the hormones your body will adjust during your pregnancy is one that may make you more prone to muscle pulls and strain.

Since your body is preparing for delivery, this hormone will loosen and relax certain ligaments and muscles, and make you more prone to injury when doing certain kinds of exercise that require balance or lifting.

Keep this in mind when you go on vacation and participate in activities you don't usually try, when you exercise, or even when you lift your toddler nephew.

You may find that your knees, legs, back and pelvis are more sensitive to strain and injury, especially during late pregnancy.

Stretch before exercise to get your muscles warmed up so you are less likely to strain them.

When you are exercising take plenty of breaks and drink a lot of water to keep you hydrated.

Try to exercise for 30 minutes, three times per week if you can.

Swimming is a great way to work out because you will be buoyant and feel light as a feather in the water, and there is no strain or jerking involved in this exercise.

Walking is also great exercise and it does not jar your joints or shins as much as jogging.

Even women who have not exercised before pregnancy, can usually begin a regimen of walking and work up to 30 minutes, three times a week on a gradual schedule.

IF you were a jogger before pregnancy, you may be able to continue this activity with some modification to schedule and intensity.

Talk to your doctor about it.

Wear good shoes and watch your balance. Remember your center of gravity has changed so you may be more prone to falls on uneven surfaces while walking or jogging.

Monitor your pulse and be sure that your heart rate does not exceed 140 beats per minute.

Do not participate in strenuous activity for more than 15 minutes at a time.

If you feel tired, overheated or dizzy, or if you get nauseous, weak or have blurred vision or heart palpitations, stop immediately and sit down and rest.

If these feelings do not pass within a few minutes after stopping the activity, call your doctor immediately.

Chapter 7: Lifestyle

Food and exercise are important components of a healthy pregnancy; so is the way you live your life.

Your lifestyle considerations include everything from the medications you take, and the amount of sleep you get, to the level of stress you experience on a daily basis.

Let's look at some of the factors you need to consider in your lifestyle:

Medication, Drugs and Medical Treatment – If you are taking prescription or over the counter medication, talk to your OB/GYN doctor about these medications and be sure you can continue taking them throughout your pregnancy.

There may be safer options you can consider, or you may have to stop taking medications, natural remedies, vitamins or supplements that are not absolutely necessary to your health during this time.

Even the most common over the counter (OTC) and pre-scription medications may be dangerous to take during pregnancy because of their effect on your unborn child.

Don't make assumptions. Talk to your doctor!

If you are seeing a specialist for a medical issue, be sure to let them know you are pregnant so that they can consider that and talk to your OB/GYN doctor if appropriate.

Remember to tell x-ray technicians and dentists that you are pregnant as well.

Ask your doctor to give you a list of 'safe over the counter medications' for things like muscle strain and headache, so you will know what to take if you need pain medication, allergy medication, etc.

As to illegal or narcotic drugs, if you are pregnant and you taking these drugs (once or frequently) you are placing your baby at risk for premature birth, birth defect, miscarriage, learning disability and lots of other things.

If you are addicted to a drug your baby can also be born addicted. Talk to your doctor about this and get help immediately.

There is no time to waste!

If you have used drugs at any time during your pregnancy, tell your doctor. Even if you stopped using the drug or didn't know you were pregnant when you used it, your baby can still be a risk and your doctor may need to monitor your pregnancy more closely.

Smoking – If you smoke and you are pregnant, get help and quit. There is no other way to say it!

Pregnant women who smoke reduce the circulation to their own bodies and to their baby, and they pass nicotine and carbon monoxide through the placenta and into the baby's body.

The risks of smoking are legendary and they have significant impact on your pregnancy, including:

- Premature birth

- Stillborn fetus

- Low birth weight stillbirth

- Sudden infant death syndrome (SIDS)

- Asthma and upper respiratory problems

Do what you have to do to quit NOW!

Sleep – You are going to need more sleep during your pregnancy and you should plan for that. Don't try to stay up until midnight to get that report done. Just give in to the fatigue and allow yourself more rest, especially during your first trimester when you are likely to feel 'bone tired'.

As your baby grows it may become difficult to find a comfortable sleep position. Most doctors recommend lying on your side with your knees bent and putting a pillow between your knees to take the strain off your lower back.

Lying on your side also makes things easier on your heart and lungs, and the baby's weight and size will not be so likely to put pressure on your blood vessels, so your legs are less likely to swell.

Sleeping on your side also helps to reduce the likelihood of varicose veins, constipation and hemorrhoids because it allows for better circulation and provides optimum blood flow to your baby and the placenta.

If you sleep on your LEFT SIDE, you are also relieving the pressure the baby's weight can put on your liver and improving blood supply to your kidneys so they can flush toxins out of your system.

Buy a few extra pillows and use them behind your back and under your stomach to give you more support.

Most stores carry full length 'body pillows', and even pregnancy pillows that are designed to support your body and your stomach.

Support and Ergonomics - If you sit a lot at work or during a commute or in a classroom, pay attention to the support you have for your back and legs during this time.

You will be sore and tired if your body is not supported appropriately.

Position your computer monitor so that the top of the screen is at or below your natural 'eye level' and elevate your feet on a stool, wastebasket or chair when you can.

Take a break every 30 minutes and walk around the office or down the hall to ask your co-worker a question. Keep moving to reduce swelling in your legs, ankles and feet and pain in your lower back.

Stress – Stress is a fact of life and it is unhealthy for everyone, but it is especially hard on you when you are pregnant and it is hard on your baby.

If your job, school or family life is stressful, if your schedule is crazy or if you are under a lot of pressure, you need to look for ways to reduce the stress.

You may have to stop working sooner if you can't find solutions at work. If your stress comes from a long or intense commute to work, consider ways to change that commute by working at home a few days a week.

Talk to your employer and your co-workers and enlist their help during the time you are pregnant. You can return the favor after you deliver.

Let your family help you with things you can afford to delegate and allow yourself to be pampered. Be willing to let things go. You don't have to vacuum every day. You can buy good take out food on occasion and ask your husband to do the laundry.

Reduce the hours you work or study and try to get more relaxation time and rest time in your schedule.

You will be better prepared for a healthy delivery if you look seriously at this issue.

Taking care of your cat – This is a great time to avoid cat litter. Pregnant women should NOT clean litter boxes, because of the risk of toxoplasmosis, spread through dirty cat litter.

Your baby may be born prematurely, suffer from poor growth or even have eye or brain damage if you are exposed to this toxic substance.

What makes this problem more serious is that you are likely to be symptom-free, while having passed toxoplasmosis to your child who child can then suffer from the effects of the toxin.

Watching your weight - You should (and will) gain weight during your pregnancy. Most of your weight gain will be during your third trimester. It is important to eat a balanced diet and exercise so that you do not gain excess weight that may hamper your recovery or your physical activity during or after pregnancy.

In general, your doctor will strive to limit your weight gain to:

- o 2-4 pounds total during the first trimester
- o 3-4 pounds per month during the second and third trimesters
- o 25-30 pounds for an average total weight gain during pregnancy*
  *if you were underweight before pregnancy: 28-40 pounds total weight gain, if you were overweight before pregnancy: 15-25 pounds total weight gain

Your total weight gain during pregnancy averages 6-8 pounds in 'baby weight', with the rest consisting of water retention, amniotic fluid, placental sac, and increased breast and uterine weight.

Of course everyone is different and weight gain depends on your personal situation, your height and your starting weight, as well. Talk to your doctor about what is right for you.

Studies have shown that women who gain more than the total recommended during pregnancy, and who do not lose this weight within six months after birth are at high risk for obesity as long as ten years after delivery.

Your doctor will monitor your weight gain at every visit and talk to you about any concerns he may have in that regard.

In the interim if you wish to monitor your weight gain and compare it against 'averages', you can find more information at this website:

http://www.verybestbaby.com/tools/trackers/mommyweight.asp?section=tl

Sex during pregnancy - Sex and pregnancy go hand in hand. But many pregnant women often have questions about sex DURING pregnancy. And sometimes pregnant women are embarrassed to ask their doctor questions about this intimate subject.

You may be concerned about whether intercourse can cause miscarriage or pose a risk to your unborn child.

Presuming you have a normal pregnancy, there is no fear of complications or problems resulting from sexual intercourse during pregnancy.

Of course you should ask your doctor about your own situation, but the average woman can and will have sex well into her third trimester.

If you start to get uncomfortable in your third trimester and it is difficult for you to achieve or sustain certain positions because of your physical size, you and your partner may want to experiment with pillows for support, or try new positions to make you more comfortable.

We don't recommend sex 'toys' during pregnancy because you don't want to introduce anything foreign that may have germs or bacteria on the surface.

Talk to your doctor about your concerns and, if you want to do some research, take a look online to find out more information and answer your specific questions.

From your first week of pregnancy to your last week of pregnancy you should consider and attend to your diet, your exercise and physical activity and lifestyle issues.

You may find it necessary to be more cautious and cease certain activities like skydiving, but in general, your pregnancy is a time when you will feel excited, healthy and NORMAL, in that you can do most anything you could do before you were pregnant.

Remember to take good care of your health so that your baby is born healthy and your delivery goes smoothly.

Most women report feeling healthy, well and happy during pregnancy.

While they may experience some discomfort as they progress through the stages of pregnancy, they are far from being invalid, and do not wish to sit in bed, or hide in the back room as their great grandmothers might have done.

For more information about exercise, diet, and lifestyle, look at these great websites:

http://www.cdc.gov/ncbddd/meds/default.htm

http://www.acog.org

http://www.cdc.gov/ncidod/nip

http://www.fns.usda.gov/fns/

http://www.cdc.gov/

http://www.ask.hrsa.gov/MCH.cfm

http://www.cdc.gov/hiv

http://www.cdc.gov/ncidol/dbmd/gbs

http://www.cdc.gov/ncidod/diseases

http://www.cdc.gov/nchstp/dstd/dstdp.htm

http://www.cdc.gov/ncbddd/fas/fasask.htm

http://www.cdc.gov/ncidod/diseases/hepatitis/index.htm

Chapter 8: The Stage of Pregnancy

Now let's look at the three stages of pregnancy and talk about how your baby develops and how your body changes during these phases so you will know how to take care of yourself and your unborn child as your pregnancy progresses.

The First Trimester

Here is what happens inside your womb during the first trimester:

Conception actually takes place about two weeks after your menstrual cycle starts. Although the 2 week period of time during and right after menstruation is counted into your 40 week gestation term, you are not actually pregnant during that time, but your doctor will calculate your due date, based on the start date of your last period.

The sperm and egg get together to form a tiny one-celled being (a zygote). The chromosomes in the zygote dictate gender, eye and hair color, height and features. After fertilization takes place, the zygote will begin to travel down the fallopian tube and into the uterus. Your little zygote is now called a 'blastocyte', a not so pretty name for your new baby.

When the blastocyte reaches the uterus it attaches itself to the uterine wall (some time between day 7 and day 9 following conception) and the placenta begins to form. *If you have been paying attention to your cycles, you may already be celebrating a positive pregnancy test by now!*

At this point, your child is officially an 'embryo' with a developing brain, spine, and organs. Not quite half way through the first trimester, your baby's heart and circulatory system will develop quickly. You won't be able to hear your baby's heart beat yet but your doctor may see the first signs of a heartbeat during an ultrasound test. Once the circulatory system has completed its circuit, the heart will beat and the first organ in your baby's body will be functional.

In week 6, your baby is about 8th of an inch in size and the neural tube for his/her brain and spine is nearly closed. The heart is beating and basic facial features are forming, including the mouth and the ears. The tissue for ribs and muscles is developing and the 'buds' are in place to grow arms and legs. Her skull is not solid yet but she has formed all the canals and channels she will need to circulate spinal fluid.

During week 8, fingers and toes are now visible, though they are still webbed. There is increased definition in the joints (ankles, elbows and wrists) and his ears lips, nose and eyelids are more defined.

By the 9th week, your baby is just about an inch long, and the embryonic 'tail' at the bottom of the spine is shrinking fast. Her head is tucked down on her chest, and she has started to form nipples, reproductive organs and hair follicles. Organs like the pancreas and gallbladder have also developed.

Nearly at the end of the first trimester, your baby has developed his vital organs, lost his embryonic tail and the webbing between his fingers and toes. His bones are form and his brain is cranking out neurons. His eyelids and his outer ears are formed and he is starting to grow 'tooth buds'

Congratulations! You now have a fetus! Genitalia is becoming apparent, and your placenta is working overtime to supply the nutrients for her growth during the 2nd and 3rd trimester.

As your first trimester draws to a close, your baby is about 3 inches long and weighs a little less than one ounce. He has fingernails and a more well defined face.

If you don't already have an OB/GYN or if you want to find another health care professional, like a midwife to follow your pregnancy, you will need to start looking for a health care provider as soon as you think you are pregnant.

Finding the best obstetrician, family doctor or nurse/midwife can be a challenge. You may wish to ask friends with children and get some personal references you trust.

Make a list of the numbers you want to call and make an appointment for a consultation so you can meet the person before you decide.

Write down the questions you want to ask and make your own decisions.

Even though references are great, you may have a different set of expectations than your neighbor.

shining armor" when things went wrong during her labor without being fully aware that her doctor's interventions, such as inducing her labor too early, may have contributed to her birthing problems in the first place).

Check with the La Leche League by calling the listing in the white pages, or looking online at www.lalecheleague.org.

They talk to pregnant and nursing women all the time and they know the local providers well.

Talk to at least three doctors or health care professionals so you know that you are choosing the one best for your style and preferences.

During the interview, ask if your health insurance will cover his/her care, ask about their experience and history delivering babies, and especially about experience with medical complications.

What hospitals or birthing centers do they attend? How often will you see them for visits and what kinds of tests will they do? How many C-sections do they perform vs. natural births? How can you reach them if you have a question or problem in between visits?

Once you have chosen your doctor or other health care professional, she/he will exam you and give you an estimated due date.

This exam may/will include blood and urine samples, a Pap smear and tests for HIV, syphilis, gonorrhea and chlamydia.

Remember that we said that your doctor will start your 'pregnancy clock' on the first day of your last menstrual cycle? You might be interested to know that the average pregnancy is 266 in length (38 weeks, not 40 weeks as calculated by your doctor).

The reason for this discrepancy is so that your doctor can take into consideration all the variables (stress, diet, variable menstrual cycles and other things).
Your doctor will give you an 'estimated due date' but if you want to figure it out for yourself you can use this calculation:

First, add 7days to the first day of your last menstrual period, then count forward 9 months. If your typical menstrual cycle is shorter or longer than 28 days, you will have to add or subtract more days to the 9 months to make the final estimated due date more accurate.

If you can't remember when your last menstrual period started, your doctor may suggest a sonogram to determine a more reasonable estimated due date, though this is not necessarily a precise way to calculate.

The fact is that when your baby is ready to be born, he/she will let you know!

A sonogram at any time during the first four months of your pregnancy can help your care provider establish your due date with a reasonable amount of accuracy, but babies' growth rates become more individual as they mature, and sonograms later on in pregnancy may not be as precise.

Less than 5% of babies arrive on the day they were predicted, so don't plan things around that day!

About one in five pregnancies results in a miscarriage, and this usually happens before the heart beat is detected. About one in eight babies arrives prematurely.

Unless there are health risks involved in a prolonged pregnancy or the bay seems to be jeopardy, your doctor will rarely suggest inducing labor. The best idea is to wait until the baby is ready.

Now that you understand your estimated due date, you will want to be sure you have all the information you need in between visits. Talk to your doctor about your diet, exercise and any medical family history you think is pertinent.

Go home! Eat right, take your prenatal vitamins, exercise and make any lifestyle changes you need to make.

If you have morning sickness, it should peak around the 8th week of your pregnancy.

Some women have more severe nausea than others, and up to 50% of pregnant women still have symptoms in their 20th week.

Other symptoms you will probably experience in your first trimester include fatigue and tenderness in your breasts.

In order to remember the things you want to discuss with your doctor at the next visit and to track dates, you may want to keep a 'pregnancy journal' and include your trimester milestones, when your next doctor's appointment is, what you have been eating and when you experienced any symptoms you want to discuss with your doctor.

If your questions are not urgent, write them down so you don't forget to ask the next time you see the doctor. If your questions or concerns are urgent, call your doctor right away.

At the end of your first trimester, your doctor may suggest a blood serum screening to determine your risk of having a baby with Down syndrome, open neural tube defect, or trisomy 18. She may also suggest a chorionic villus sampling if you have a family history of genetic problems. If your doctor suggests other tests, ask him why he is re-commending these tests and what the results will tell him.

If test results are not good, remember that your doctor has more options and remedies for problem pregnancies than ever before in history. Get all the information about the issue and remain calm. Your doctor may suggest you see a specialist if her concerns are serious.

Finally, a word about pregnancy-related headaches. These can come from hormonal changes, dehydration and lots of other sources.

If you experience a migraine headache during pregnancy, know that about 15% of pregnant women get migraines during this time, and it is usually during early pregnancy.

About 10-30 minutes before onset of a migraine, you may start to feel tired and nauseated. You may even get blurred vision or see tiny points of flashing light. Other symptoms can include a tingling sensation in your hands or legs and sensitivity to light and sound.

Ask your doctor how to treat these headaches and understand that they usually go away as your pregnancy progresses.

If your headache includes any of the following symptoms, call your doctor immediately: sudden or explosive head pain, headache accompanied by fever and/or stiff neck, headaches accompanied by slurred speech or serious vision problems.

If you work in a strenuous job or in a risky environment, you should tell your employer about your pregnancy immediately and talk to your doctor about taking your leave sooner or see if you can work in another section of the company temporarily.

An example of a risky job might be a job where you have to climb or balance (like a telephone repair job), a chemist, x-ray technician, medical disease research, or a job where you have to do a lot of lifting, or a job where you work in a poorly ventilated location, or where it is very hot or very cold all the time.

You should also be wary of jobs that require you to travel to countries where you might be exposed to exotic or contagious diseases.

The Second Trimester

What's happening inside the womb now:

Your baby is more active, though you can't quite feel it moving yet. He may start to put his thumb in his mouth now, and his skull is starting to get more solid. Ribs are starting to form but aren't quite visible yet.

Early in the second trimester, hormones are having their effect! The prostate gland or ovaries are developing. The roof of your baby's mouth is nearly complete.

Around the third week of this trimester, your baby now has a layer of transparent skin, and is starting to form eyebrows and hair on his head. Eyes and ears have more definition and bone and marrow are now forming.

One month into the 2nd trimester, your child is four and five inches in length and weighs nearly 3 ounces. Your baby's eyes are becoming sensitive to light. Her eyes are becoming sensitive to light and she can squint, frown and display other expressions. She can also make a fist.

That all important fat layer that keeps us warm and protects and energizes our body is forming now. Your child can swallow! The nerves in his brain are now connected to the ears which have reached their final position on the skull. Your son can hear your heart beat, and the rumble of hunger in your stomach. He may react to loud noises outside his environment but jumping or moving.

By the 18th week of your pregnancy, you may already have felt the first signs of life in your womb. If not, you WILL soon. Your baby's hearing has improved. He can faintly hear your voice and the voices of others as you converse. He can move his muscles reflexively and his kidneys are producing urine which is stored in your amniotic sac after it is excreted. He has a new coating (vernix) and very fine hair (lanugo) to protect his thin skin.

About 6 inches long now, weighing about 9 ounces your baby is most likely moving around by now and you can feel it! Her skin is thicker and less transparent and she has eyebrows and some hair on her head. During this trimester, bone marrow begins to produce blood cells and your child starts to ingest sugar from your amniotic fluid.

Your baby is about one pound around 21 weeks into your pregnancy. She has developed a sense of touch and now has taste buds. Genitalia is complete.

Your child will practice breathing by moving your amniotic fluid in and out of his lungs. His skin is much less transparent and he is developing more fat.

Your son has fingerprints! His inner ear has developed to the point where he can sense whether he is upside down in the womb. By now, he will have developed a schedule or cycle for sleep and wakefulness

Fingers and hands are fully developed though your baby's ability to control these tools is far from refined. You will notice more movement as your child explores his limited universe within the womb.

Maybe close to 2 pounds by your 25th week, your baby is growing faster with clearly defined eyebrows, eyelashes and eyes. At the end of this trimester, you are 2/3 of the way to delivery and the changes you and your baby experience during the final trimester will be even more dramatic. Right now your baby's organs and immune system are working hard to reach completion in time for delivery, and he has grown to 3-4 times in length since the end of the first trimester.

During your second trimester you may still be experiencing morning sickness and you may have started to have headaches and a sensitivity and aversion to certain smells and foods.

If you have waited to tell your family, co-workers and friends about your pregnancy, you can probably do so now. Most women are skittish about announcing a pregnancy before the second trimester begins because miscarriage most often occurs during the first trimester.

If your appearance or your symptoms changed early in your pregnancy, you may already have been faced with this announcement.

If you work in a risky job or a strenuous or dangerous position, you have probably already told your employer you are pregnancy and decided on what you will do to protect your child and yourself during your pregnancy. If you have NOT done this, you need to do it ASAP.

During this trimester you will want to start thinking about and talking to your doctor about delivery-related issues.

Give yourself plenty of time to talk about these things and decide so you are not caught short when you are trying to prepare your home and family for the impending delivery during your first trimester.

Where will you have the baby, who will you choose as your pediatrician? Will you take childbirth classes and have a natural delivery or do you want to opt for pain medication during birth.

If you are going to take a childbirth course, ask your doctor for recommendations and remember that you will usually need a partner.

You can also find out about the alternatives by looking on these websites:

http://www.lamaze.org

http://www.braleybirth.com

Another question you might discuss with your doctor is whether to breast feed or use formula?

As long as we are on the topic of breast feeding, let's talk about the changes in your breasts and how to best care for your breasts during pregnancy and prepare them for breast feeding, if that is your choice.

Your breasts are going to get bigger over the course of your pregnancy, and your rib cage will get wider to accommodate your growing baby.

You may notice tiny blue blood vessels on your chest as your blood vessels dilate and enlarge.
Your nipples and areola (the dark area surrounding the nipple) will get larger and darker so that your newborn infant can more easily see them for nursing after birth.

Little bump may appear around your areola. These are oil glands that help to keep the area around your nipples clean for nursing.

Sometime around your 14th week of pregnancy, your nipples will start to leak a whitish fluid called 'colostrum'; a rich protein-filled form of early milk that will clear your child's digestive tract after delivery.

You can buy disposable breast to absorb leaks and keep your skin from getting irritated. Tuck them inside your bra and avoid embarrassing leaks!

Be sure you purchase a roomier bra to accommodate your enlarged breasts. You can consider wearing a nursing bra if you'd like. They are comfortable and have a lot of cushioning and stretch. To take care of your breasts as they change, consider these suggestions:

Use clear water to rinse your breasts when bathing so that the protective oils produced by the new oil glands are not washed away.

If you want to toughen your nipples to make the nursing transition easier and less painful, you can use a soft washcloth to rub them so that they get tougher. As you adjust to this texture, you can graduate to something rougher so that your nipples are not quite as sensitive by the time you start to nurse your baby.

If your breasts are swollen or uncomfortable, you can put a cool ice pack inside a wash cloth and hold it against the side of the breast to bring down the swelling or take a warm shower to soothe the tissue.

During your second trimester, your doctor may recommend other tests to monitor the growth of your baby.

Amniocentesis is usually performed between 13 and 18 weeks, sometimes later in the pregnancy depending on the situation. The doctor will numb your abdomen and insert a long needle into the amniotic sac. There is no risk to your baby.
The fluid drawn from the sac can tell the doctor about abnormalities or problems. If you are over 35, your doctor may recommend this test to be sure that your pregnancy is progressing normally.

A percutaneous umbilical blood sampling (PUBS, or cordiocentesis) helps your doctor tell if your baby suffers from specific diseases like sickle cell disease and hemophilia. In this test, a needle is also passed through your abdomen, into your uterus.

But in this case, the doctor will draw a small sample of blood from the umbilical cord.

Some time around week 15 of your pregnancy your doctor may suggest an ultrasound or sonogram, to look at the size of your baby and determine whether your pregnancy is on schedule.

An ultrasound is painless, but you do have drink and hold a lot of water, so you may be a bit uncomfortable. The technician will use a handheld device and slide it back and forth across your abdomen, to produce an image of your baby from high frequency sound waves.

If you are still exercising by the end of your 2nd trimester – good for you!

Just remember not to push yourself until you are out of breath or exhausted. Take breaks and allow yourself the luxury of adjusting to your new size and shape.

Avoid exercise that strains your lower back or legs, or exercises that require you to lie flat on the floor.

Instead of riding a bike in the street, consider riding a stationary bike so that your balance and shifting center of gravity do not cause you to fall.

You can exercise by scrubbing the floor or taking a power walk to the post office or corner market.

This is also a good time to start your Kegel exercises, named after Dr. Arnold Kegel. Kegel exercises strengthen your pelvic floor and prepare you for delivery, and you can do them anywhere.

Tighten and release the muscles on your pelvic floor as if you were trying to stop the flow of urine.

The name of the muscle you are tightening and releasing is 'pubococcygeus' (PC) and it goes from your pubic bone to your tailbone. Pregnancy can weaken this muscle and cause you to leak urine when you laugh, cough or strain.

One study reported that 50% of pregnant women had symptoms of 'bladder weakness' during and after pregnancy.

But the Kegel exercise doesn't just keep you dry, it keeps your baby's head in the best position for labor and delivery, so it is doubly important.

Don't make the mistake of tightening your entire lower abdomen, thighs and/or buttocks. Be sure you isolate and specify the muscle by thinking of tightening the muscle you would tighten to stop urinating.

Kegel is easy to do, and you can do it whenever you THINK about doing it; at the grocery store or at work. Start with 10 to 25 cycles, a few times a day, and work your way up to 100 squeezes a day.

Sometime during this trimester, you will probably notice a change in your hair and skin texture. Some women report oilier or drier than normal hair and skin, and some even say their hair gets straighter or curlier.

Some women also report that their hair grows faster, and that their skin is more sensitive when they are pregnant.

The glands that produce oil in your body will increase or decrease production depending on your hormonal balance.

For some women, the second trimester of their pregnancy signals the best 'hair days' of their lives.

While there is no evidence that coloring your hair can hurt your baby, if you want to stay away from harsh dyes or permanent solutions you can ask your stylist to use techniques that do not directly impact the scalp and provide only highlights or temporary color.

But remember that your new hair texture may 'take' dye in a different way than your old hair once did. So, be ready for anything!

This is the time most women buy a new pair of larger shoes. Yes, your feet do grow during pregnancy and may grow as much as one full size. Choose comfortable, slip on, supportive shoes and wear maternity pantyhose if you find your legs getting tired or swollen during the day.

Sometime between week 18 and week 22 of your pregnancy you will feel your baby moving in the womb.

If you are overweight it may take longer for you to feel movement. And sometimes the placenta is located toward the front of the uterus so it is harder to feel the baby move until it gets larger.

In time your baby will kick and move and the feeling will be so sharp that it is hard to ignore. By the 23rd week, your baby is much more sensitive to sound and touch coming from the outside so you can expect that you will get a response if something startling happens.

A baby's activity will increase up to 10 times the normal level when mom is under emotional stress. So if you have a near miss car accident or something startles you, you will notice your baby's reaction, a well.

Pregnancy hormones will also act on your emotions so be prepared to feel overly emotional about everyday things and to have some strange and emotional dreams when you sleep. This is all normal. However, IF you experience any signs of depression or mental disturbance, be sure to talk to your doctor immediately.

In general, the second trimester will be easier than the first and the third. By now you are used to coping with heartburn, back pain, headaches, fatigue and other symptoms and you have adjusted your lifestyle to accommodate your pregnancy.

Be sure to drink plenty of water, eat right, keep your blood sugar in check and get plenty of rest. If you work or go to school, be sure to get your feet up as often as possible to keep your back and legs from bothering you.

The Third Trimester

15 inches long, weighing between 2 and 3 pounds, your baby is now opening and closing her eyes. He sleeps for about 20-30 minutes at a stretch. He is becoming rather athletic and some of his kicks may take your breath away! His bones are still flexible but getting stronger every day.

Practice breathing is taking place inside the womb as your baby practices for the real world outside. You may feel tiny jerks and twitches if your baby gets the hiccups during practice.   While the lungs are not fully developed, they are getting closer. Babies born at this point in pregnancy can survive but would probably be on a ventilator.

Your baby's protective coating of hair (lanugo) will start to disappear, and her lungs are nearly fully developed. Her pupils are functional and will constrict and dilate when exposed to light and dark.

Your baby is gaining weight more rapidly now as he adds fat to his body to prepare for the rigors of birth and the outside world. You will feel lots of stretching, kicking and rolling now!

At about 36 weeks into your pregnancy, your child is approximately 6 pounds and 18 inches long, and is practicing sucking in preparation for nursing in the real world. If you are on target for delivery, your baby may 'flip' this week and turn over into the 'heads down' position for birth.

Anytime now! If you deliver during the next few weeks, you are pretty average in terms of the length of your pregnancy. Every week you continue to carry your child, she will gain more weight in the womb and get stronger though she is running out of room to play so her activity and kicking may seem to slow down.

At 38 weeks, if you have not delivered, your baby is nearly 7 pounds. Did you know that your baby's brain and nervous system are still developing, and WILL throughout his childhood and well into adolescence? Now that your baby has finished storing fat, his body temperature will hold stable when he is born. And the antibodies he receives through your placenta will help him get through the first few months after birth in good health.

At 40 weeks, if you haven't delivered yet, your baby will probably be about 7 or 8 pounds and around 20 inches at birth. Don't be too concerned if your due date passes without labor. Only about 5% of pregnant women delivery on their due dates and your doctor will probably not recommend induction for a week or two after you are due, unless you or your baby are in jeopardy.

As you pass through your third trimester, your body is changing more quickly.

Nearly all pregnant women get stretch marks, those streaks that appear on your stomach and thighs as your body expends.

There is no 'cure' for stretch marks, but they do fade after pregnancy.

Keep your skin hydrated by drinking plenty of water and use a good non-greasy moisturizer on your abdomen, and legs to prevent dryness and keep the worst of the stretch marks at bay. This moisturizing will also decrease itching which many pregnant women report during late pregnancy.

You may also see varicose or spider veins during your late pregnancy. These most commonly appear around your ankles and feet where you have lots of swelling, but they can appear in other places as well.

Wear maternity pantyhose and put your feet up often to reduce swelling.

If you find that you perspire more easily, use powder and wear well-ventilated clothing so that you don't get a rash or increase perspiration and odor during these late months.

About one in 150 women encounter pruritic urticarial papules (PUPP) during late pregnancy. These are red, itchy patches that usually appear on your stomach. Talk to your doctor to get a good cream to treat these patches.

Be careful not to get overheated or hold your breath for long periods of time when you are in late pregnancy. This will affect the blood vessels in your body which are already working overtime to provide oxygenated blood to you and to your baby.

Every woman complains about sagging breasts in late pregnancy and after pregnancy but you should know that gravity will take its toll even if you never had a child.

So relax!

There is no way, short of surgery, to make your breasts small and perky again but you should acknowledge the changes by wearing a supportive bra, and you can help yourself by using good poster and by lifting arm weights and doing arm exercises to give your chest muscles more tone.

You will want to wait until after you deliver to do this, though!

As your baby grows to about 28 weeks in the womb, she/he will run out of room to play and kick and you may notice a bit less activity. Someplace around week 35 or 36, your baby will turn into the 'heads down' position for birth and you may notice that the bulge in your abdomen 'drops' lower.

This will put even more pressure on your bladder and you will feel like you are running to the bathroom every five minutes, though you will welcome the relief of pressure on your rib cage.

Though your baby's movement has slowed, you should still feel the baby moving about 10 times within a 2 hr period.

If you do not feel movement during a reasonably long time period and you are concerned, call your doctor immediately.

But be aware that there may be no problem. Your baby may be sleeping during that time. If your doctor feels the need to monitor your child, he may suggest a non-stress test to determine the baby's heart rate and ensure that the baby is not in any distress.

During your late pregnancy, your doctor may advise a urine test or a glucose tolerance test if you have a family history of diabetes or if your blood sugar has been high.

In these last few months you may notice more problems with digestion and heartburn, simply because there is less space for your body to do its work.

Be sure to drink plenty of water and try to eat small amounts more often so you are not overstuffed. Take a walk after you eat to stimulate digestion.

Some pregnant women sleep in a 'propped' position or support themselves with pillows to allow better digestion and to relieve discomfort.

During your last weeks of pregnancy you will probably align your sleep patterns to those of your baby. By now, you are hopefully on maternity leave and if you have difficulty getting enough rest, you may want to try to nap when you feel the need.

Your baby is likely to squirm when you lie down. This is because he can adjust and take a bit more space for himself when you are lying down, so let him get comfortable after you get comfortable.

In order to improve your sleep, eat a light meal at dinner time so you don't feel stuffed, and try taking a walk after dinner.

Take a warm (not extremely hot) bath before bed and stretch a little to loosen your muscles. Listen to relaxing music and be sure the room is dark so you can sleep.

It is common for pregnant women to experience painless Braxton-Hicks contractions during the last few months of pregnancy. These do not signal labor, but instead will fade and disappear.

Some changes you WILL note that indicate you are getting closer:

Your doctor may report that your cervix is thinner and is starting to dilate. This doesn't mean you are going to the hospital at that moment, though. You may wait for a few days before it is time.

You may see a small amount of pink or red jelly-like stain indicated that the plug that seals off the mouth of the uterus has come loose. Labor may still be a few days off but let your doctor know that this has happened.

Remember that your baby will give your body the signal when he/she is ready to be born. A complex set of hormonal changes will take place to soften the cervix and start contractions that will push the baby out into the world.

If you go well beyond your due date, your doctor may suggest keeping a 'kick count' to see how active your baby is over a certain number of hours. Or he may suggest a sonogram to measure amniotic fluid, and fetal activity.

If you are past 40 weeks gestation, your doctor MAY suggest that you induce labor, though most doctors prefer to wait for the baby's signal. However, if your baby is in distress or if your pregnancy is protracted and causing you health problems, induction may be necessary.

Your doctor will check you into the hospital and give you medication to start or enhance contractions and to get the process moving.

Chapter 9: Be Prepared - Planning for Delivery

During your second or third trimester, you should begin to look at the hospitals or birthing centers with whom your health care professional is associated.

If you have a choice of facilities, take a tour of the maternity area to decide which facility you prefer. You can arrange a tour by calling the hospital or birthing center.

We'll give you some suggestions on questions to ask and things to look for that will make your delivery day easier and ensure that there are no surprises.

Patient's Rights and Informed Consent – Remember that you have rights as a patient and get a copy of the hospital or birthing center privacy and patient rights brochures. Read it thoroughly and be sure to ask your doctor and the staff at the facility any questions you may have about these standards.

Any medical procedures, tests, medications or other action that is administered to you during your delivery and your time in the hospital requires 'informed consent'.

In other words, the staff must explain what they are doing and WHY they are doing it and you have the right to refuse treatment if you wish.

You doctor, midwife and medical staff MUST tell you about the benefits AND the risks of any procedure or action they plan to take.

The consent form you sign when you are admitted does not mean you can't change your mind about a specific procedure or issue, so ask questions and know your rights.

Understand that your doctor is bound by oath and by law to care for you and your baby so if you refuse a procedure that she feels is necessary she may choose to proceed with this procedure anyway and she is legally protected if she does so. You will have to sort out the legality and the outcome after delivery!

You also have a right to ask for a second opinion about your treatment but in an emergency, there may not be time to call for another doctor and get that second opinion.

It is important to note that, in most cases, your pregnancy and delivery will proceed in a healthy manner and you will never be faced with these kinds of life and death decisions.

But, even for the small decisions where you have options, you do have the right to get a second opinion or to refuse what your doctor recommends, so it is important that you know your rights. Your doctor, midwife and medical staff are there to help you, not to hurt you, and in most cases, you won't face any significant disagreement.

Once you have chosen your birthing facility, get familiar with the procedures and the layout of the facility so that you can relax and be calm on the day of your delivery.

Remember, if you know where you are going and what is going to happen to you, you are less likely to be stressed over the small details.

And you will need your energy and focus to attend to your labor and delivery.

Things to Know about the Maternity Care Facility - If you are going to write a 'birth plan' that indicates your wishes for how you want your labor and delivery managed, ask to have this plan put on file and find out whether you need to bring another copy when you come to the hospital (just in case they can't find the one you gave them).

We'll give you some details about drafting a birth plan in a minute.

Also, find out if they will FOLLOW this plan, presuming there are no emergencies or special circumstances. Does your chosen hospital have policies they must follow for all patients in labor? If so, you should find out what they are so that you can take them into consideration when you write your birth plan.

Find out about nursing care as well. How many nurses are on duty in the birthing center or maternity area? How long are their shifts? How many patients does each nurse manage?

Ask about birth-related statistics: How many babies are delivered at this facility per year? How many are vaginal births (with or without medication), how many are C-sections?

How many births do they induce every year (*be sure you talk to your doctor about his/her policies in this regard as well, so that you know you will be allowed ample opportunity to delivery before he recommends an induction*).

Ask whether your hospital or facility is a teaching hospital where you may have students or residents treating you. If so, and if you are not comfortable with this, find out if you can refuse treatment by students and residents and how to do that, if necessary.

And ask how you will have to request a second opinion if you need one.
What devices does your hospital use to monitor your labor and your baby's progress during labor?   Does this facility use continuous electronic fetal monitoring?

If don't want this monitoring on a continuous basis, do you have the option of periodic monitoring?

If you are uncomfortable during labor and wish to refuse a pelvic exam, can you do so?

Does the birthing center or maternity wing have an obstetrical anesthesiologist on call in case you need one? Can you make an appointment to talk to an anesthesiologist before you go into labor so that you understand your options for pain medication and what will happen if you need a C-section?

Be sure you ask the anesthesiologist to explain the use of an epidural. What is it, how is it administered and how will it effect you during and after delivery? When is the epidural administered during labor? Is it always effective?

Talk to the staff and the anesthesiologist about the procedures for C-sections. How and when will the decision be made? Will your labor coach or partner be allowed to stay in the operating room with you?

Where is the procedure performed? Can you see the room in advance so you know what to expect? Where will you be moved after surgery and how long will stay in the recovery area? What kind of medication will they give you for pain?

Will you have IVs or a catheter and if so, when will they be removed? How will this procedure effect your ability to nurse and take care of your baby?

Prepare for Your Time After the Baby is Born - Take a tour of the nursery and find out if your baby will be allowed to stay in your room most of the day or if she/he will be brought to you at certain hours for feeding. What if you are not feeling well? Will the baby stay in the nursery temporarily or will the baby stay in your room?

Ask about special care facilities for your newborn. What if your baby is born prematurely or has a medical problem? Where is this special nursery? Can you take a tour of the facility and see what the equipment and nursing staff is like?

Neonatal Intensive Care Units (NICU) are very important if you have a child with special needs, so be sure you understand your options in this regard.

What is the visiting policy? Can you visit your baby at any time? Will you need to wear special gowns or clothing to go into the room?

Get a list of the routine vaccinations and procedures they plan for your baby: injections, tests, medications, etc.

And ask what each of these means so that you know what they are doing when the staff tells you they are about to perform a test or give your baby a shot.

If you have a boy, ask about the hospital policy regarding circumcision. Is this optional or do they automatically circumcise your child. Will your child receive pain medication for the circumcision and afterwards if necessary? If you are Jewish and you plan to have this done by a *moile*, be sure to let the hospital know this!

Lastly, find out how long your hospital stay will be for a normal vaginal delivery and for a C-section birth if required.

Now, take all these details and consider them for your birth plan. Make it specific so that your doctor and medical staff don't have to guess if you are unable to discuss it with them.

The reason we suggest a birth plan is because it helps you to organize and consider your preferences and to ask all the right questions of your doctor and your hospital or birthing center staff so you are well prepared for your delivery.

Birth plans are not legal documents, but you should show yours to your doctor and get him to sign off on your plans to be sure you are being reasonable in your expectations.

Include information in your birth plan about whether you want induction, amniocentesis, IVs, heparin locks, enemas, epidurals, medications or narcotics, whether you want to eat or drink, use a birthing tub, move around or walk during labor, how you wish to be monitored (continuous or periodic), whether you want your doctor to use forceps, whether you want 'self-directed' pushing vs. doctor directed pushing.

Keep your birth plan short and easy to read (try to type it if you can so no one has to struggle over poor hand writing). Hospital staff will not read the document if it is too long and wordy. Describe what you want and what you don't want!

Your birth plan can also include what happens after delivery: Do want your husband to cut the umbilical cord, and hold the baby first? Will your baby receive medication or vaccine, will she be breast fed or bottle fed? What happens if your baby needs special care?

When you think about what you want and what you don't want you are more likely to talk to your doctor about all the crucial requirements before you get to the hospital. And there is often no time to have this discussion during labor.

Birth plans *can* have disadvantages. Some doctors and medical staff do not appreciate being told what you want, but in that case, you may be using the wrong staff.

If you have a 'testy' health care professional on your hands – but one you would like to keep because of their knowledge and skills – be prudent about how you approach your birth plan.

Talk to them first about the fact that you are thinking of doing one and ask for their input. That will get them engaged. After you've done the birth plan ask them to look at it and give you feedback.

Be willing to be flexible and reasonable. Don't feel you have to control every detail. Most doctors and hospital staff are reasonable enough to work with you if you approach them in a polite and respectful manner.

Now that you have drafted your birth plan, there are a few other things you'll want to ask your hospital or birthing center staff to be prepared for going home with your baby.

Ask if your birthing center or hospital offers 'after care' visits from nurses, lactation consultants or other health care professionals after you have been discharged from the facility.

And be sure you find out about classes or support groups for new parents. Most facilities offer these on site and others will recommend a community-based program that will help you learn basic skills like bathing your infant.

Some groups, like the La Leche League, provide support for nursing mothers.

And there are even support group round tables where new parents can share their excitement and concerns with other new parents and get answers from a skilled, knowledgeable facilitator.

Chapter 10: The Big Day is Finally Here - What to do During Labor

The waiting is over. You have finally reached the big day!

You should know that only about one in ten pregnant women experiences the legendary 'breaking of the waters' as a first sign of impending birth.

If you are one of those women, you may feel a slow trickle that is only enough to dampen your underwear, or you may wake up to a wet sheet in the morning. Rarely is there a dramatic gush of water.

The water from your amniotic sac has a slightly salty smell and it is clear and a bit sticky with some flecks. If your amniotic fluid is cloudy or green, tell your doctor this.

Labor contractions do not start right away, but they will usually appear somewhere between 24 and 48 hours after your amniotic fluid is released.

In any case, you should call your doctor to let him know that your 'water has broken'.

He will probably want you to come into the office for a visit so he can determine where you are in your labor schedule. He will probably apply an antiseptic cream around the opening to your uterus to be sure that you have protection against infection until your baby is born.

While you are waiting for your contractions to start, take showers, *not baths*, and don't allow anything into your vagina other than your doctor's sterile glove!

Before you go into you may have some diarrhea or vomiting. This doesn't always happen but it will happen in many women. If you do experience these symptoms, your labor will typically begin within 12-24 hrs after the onset of nausea or diarrhea.

DO NOT try any herbal remedies or other things to induce labor on your own!

The following symptoms do not signal labor but may indicate a medical problem. You should call your doctor immediately if you experience any of these:

- o Abdominal pain as opposed to uterine pain
- o Vaginal bleeding
- o Absence of fetal movement for 24 hours (after the fifth month of your pregnancy)
- o Dim or blurry vision, or severe or constant headache
- o Severe swelling of eyelids, hands or face during last trimester
- o Persistent, severe vomiting

When your labor starts, you will know that you are not having the old standby Braxton Hicks contractions you have had during your pregnancy.

Remember that these contractions are relatively painless and last only 30-60 seconds. True labor contractions are longer and more regular and will not go away.

They will increase in strength and severity as your labor progresses and they will get closer together as your delivery draws near.

You don't have to run to the hospital or birthing center at the first sign of labor. You are more likely to remain calm and comfortable at home and you will usually have plenty of time to get there.

If your partner or labor coach is at a distance from you or the hospital, let them know you have started labor and get someone to sit with you for awhile if it will make you make comfortable.

Allow plenty of time to get to the hospital if you live in a city or if you are leaving around rush hour.

If this is your first baby you may find that you are more un-comfortable during the first part of labor than during the last part. For experienced mothers, the end of the labor cycle seems to be more difficult. Whatever the case, don't panic. If you have taken a course for natural childbirth, you don't have to start your breathing and child birth strategies right away.

Just relax and wait until you need them!

You may have another 10 or 12 hours before you deliver and you want to you're your strength for the final sprint. Rest and drink plenty of water. You can even eat a little if you find you have an appetite. Just don't overload your stomach.

Eat healthy food like protein and vegetables or whole grain bread or just nibble on crackers and fruit.

If you find you want to take a bath be sure you have help to get you in and out of the tub at home!

You should contact your doctor to let them know that labor has started.

She will probably tell you to call back when your con-tracts are about one minute in length and about five minutes apart.

If you are still not sure whether your labor is 'real', give yourself this mental test:

False Labor (prodromal) or Braxton-Hicks Contractions –
Remember that Braxton- Hicks contractions stay at about
the same intensity over the time have them. They are the
same an hour ago as they are now and they only last 30
seconds or so.

These contractions will go away if you walk, move or
change positions. There is no significant discomfort or
pain associated with these contractions. You may have a
backache.

The less common 'prodromal labor, is a kind of 'dry run' or
practice labor that can cause lower back pain with contractions.

These contractions may feel more real than Braxton-Hicks,
but they will not get closer together or stronger over time.
If you get up and move around they will sometimes disappear completely.

Labor Contractions – Get progressively stronger and last
longer as the hours go by. They also get closer together as
your labor progresses.

There is significant discomfort with these contractions, and nothing you do seems to change that. You can move, walk or change positions and the contractions are still strong and predictable and painful.

You have pain in the back and in your abdomen (like a 'too tight' seatbelt or band around your stomach that keeps getting tighter).

IMPORTANT: *If at any time you feel a significant pressure to push, you should get to the hospital immediately, and forget the leisurely labor at home! If you can feel a bulge or firm protrusion between your legs at the mouth of your cervix, you should not try to make it to the hospital. Have someone call 911 and get yourself comfortable on your bed with extra clean towels or a clean (old) comforter underneath you. Or, if you are more comfortable on the floor, be sure you have plenty of clean padding underneath you and relax and breathe until the ambulance and EMTs arrive.*

When you are ready to go to the hospital, don't try to go alone if you can help it. Have someone take you, call a cab or call an ambulance if you must.

When you get to the hospital on the day of delivery, be sure you ask if they have a copy of the birth plan. If not, have another copy ready to give them, *and repeat your primary and most important requests then and there* so that you remind the staff of what you want.

During labor your cervix will become thinner and more open. If you are a first time mother, this may take 10 hours or more. If you have already had a child it may take only 2-3 hours. Your doctor will refer to this dual process as 'effacing' and 'dilating', and he will use your progress to determine how soon you may give birth.

The thinning of the cervix (effacement), is noted as a percentage. If you are 25% effaced, you are only ¼ of the way there.

The widening of the opening in your cervix (dilation) is noted in centimeters or sometimes in 'fingers'. When your cervix is fully dilated it is about 10 centimeters across.

Or your doctor may say you are '2 or 3 fingers' dilated, meaning your cervix is dilated by about 3-4 centimeters and still has a way to go.

As your labor progresses, contractions will get more intense and you will have shorter breaks between these contractions. But even at the longest point of your labor, these contractions never last more than 1.5 min. and you will typically have at least 30 sec between contractions.

Each contraction occurs in three stages:

- The Increment Phase (or start-up)
- The Acme Phase (the height of the contraction)
- The Decrement Phase (the contraction slows to a halt)

And you will get a brief rest in between each cycle.

The discomfort of labor is primarily from the pressure and weight of the baby's body putting pressure on your organs and body and traveling down through the birth canal, causing the hips to widen and the head and body to push against the cervix.

Stage 1 Labor - The upper half of your uterus becomes more dense and the lower half thinner so that it push against your baby to propel him/her down into the birth canal. Every time you have a contraction during this stage, your baby will move down and then come back up a little as it progresses through the narrow change in your pelvis.

Stage 2 Labor – Begins as soon as your cervix and uterus have completed their effacing and dilation processes. This stage is considerably shorter than the first stage and may last 20-60 minutes. Unless you are heavily medicated or you have had an epidural, she will feel like you MUST start pushing your baby out.

Try to resist this urge unless and until your doctor tells you to go ahead. And if you are going to push, try to control the 'when' on your own schedule, gently pushing with breathing in between so that you can go with what your body is telling you to do.

Because the uterus does most of the work, you may not have to push much at all and what doctors call the 'valsalv maneuver' or the 'purple push' will raise your blood pressure and tire you more quickly.

So, if your doctor asks you to push, ask him to do it on your own count as you are ready. Your baby will born within the same time period and you and the baby will both be less stressed.

Once your baby is born your doctor will snip the umbilical cord (the umbilical cord is about 22 inches long, and looks rather like a spiral tube with a white membrane covering it), and your baby will become its own independent entity, no longer dependent on your body though certainly dependent on you as her new mother in this brave new world!

The doctor will then take the baby for a moment to clean out her mouth and record her vital statistics (weight, length, etc.). You will probably get a chance to hold the baby right after he has finished his work.

Remember that babies arrive on their own schedule, so your labor may be shorter or longer than someone else's. In most cases, this is just what is normal for you and for THIS baby – not necessarily what will happen in any subsequent births.

Before we finish talking about labor, we should note that you have one more thing to do before your delivery is over.

You have to expel the placenta (the amniotic sac that has nourished and cradled your baby while he/she has developed in your uterus).

During your pregnancy, the placenta is attached to the wall of your uterus with slender threads or roots and it gets its nourishment for your baby from your body.

It stores carbohydrates, minerals, protein, and fats and feeds them to your child through the umbilical cord, and it is the conduit for oxygen to your baby's body.

It also carries away waste matter and carbon monoxide which is then washed through your kidneys and out of your system.

At the time of your baby's birth, the placenta will be about 6-8 inches in diameter, about 1 inch thick and about one pound in weight.

After your baby is born, the placenta will detach itself from the uterine wall so you can 'deliver' it through the same channel from which your baby was born.

If you see the placenta while your doctor is delivering it, you will notice its rich red, kidney bean color and a texture that is squishy and sponge-like.

Your doctor will put the placenta in a bowl and examine it to be sure that it is intact and there are no fragments missing that may still be attached to the uterine wall.

Within hours after delivery, your uterus will shrink, reverting to almost normal size within ten days after your baby is born.

For about six weeks after delivery, you will experience some bleeding as your uterus cleans out the remaining fluid and other artifacts of your pregnancy. If this discharge has a foul or strange odor, call your doctor and let her know.

A few months after 'house keeping' activities are completed, your ovaries will release another egg, and you are once again ready to 'make a baby'.

Chapter 11: Summary

Giving birth is indeed a strange and wonderful thing. It is a very natural event and should not be considered an 'illness' though you may need medication or surgery in some instances.

Still, with all the knowledge doctors, midwives and nurses have about pregnancy and birth, every mother and every child is different. Every pregnancy is different and every labor and delivery is different.

No matter how much research you do and no matter how much you want to control your pregnancy and delivery, your baby always seems to have a mind of its own when it comes to how it will develop and when it will make its appearance.

Many new mothers look back on their pregnancy and delivery and wonder if they could have done something differently.

Should you have chosen a different OB/GYN doctor, pediatrician or hospital? Did you go to the hospital in time? Should you have decided to breast feed instead of using a bottle?

Hindsight may be 20/20 but you should understand that pregnancy and delivery are probably the last things you should try to *control* in your life.

You can and should take good care of yourself and your baby, but there is a lot left to nature in this process.

Birth is a profound and mysterious process and no matter how good your medical care, no matter how careful you are, in the end, it is up to nature to do its job.

If you find yourself worrying over these things after your baby is born, talk to your doctor and your family about what you are feeling.

Remember that it is normal to want to do the best you can for your child and you are likely to be your own harshest judge.

Put things in perspective!

For much of our societal history babies were born at home, or even in fields or by the side of the road. And we managed to deliver healthy children who lived to a ripe old age.

Today, 97% of our babies are delivered in hospitals by OB/GYN doctors.

The best advice we can give you for your pregnancy AND post partum time after you bring your baby home is to be flexible and calm.

Don't be too quick to panic or become concerned, but be sensitive to the changes in your body and talk to your doctor if you are worried about any symptom or issue.

Give your baby the best chance at starting life healthy by eating right, exercising and making any necessary life style changes.

We haven't had any time to talk about work or travel, but be smart when you consider how long you will continue to work or when/if you are going to travel in late pregnancy.

Don't push yourself, especially if the job you have is risky or strenuous.

On average you have an EXCELLENT chance of delivery a healthy, happy baby so enjoy your pregnancy and get all the rest you can.

You will need it after that little bundle of joy enters your life!

Warmest regards,

Martha Diebold

RESOURCES

You have at your fingertips valuable information designed to help you with your pregnancy. The internet is a rich source of information that you can access anywhere in the world.

This is also part and parcel of being empowered with information so that you can make better informed decisions for yourself.

Because information changes at the speed of light you will have access to the latest cutting edge information when it comes to hand.

Here are some helpful resources you may find useful.

Glossary:

http://www.happyhealthypregnancy.com/info/pregnancy_tools/preg_terms.aspx

You can also find out about the birth alternatives by looking on these websites:

http://www.lamaze.org
http://www.braleybirth.com

If you need more information on mercury levels in fish, use this website:

http://www.cfsan.fda.gov/~frf/sea-mehg.html

For more information about exercise, diet, and lifestyle, look at these great websites:

http://www.cdc.gov/ncbddd/meds/default.htm

http://www.acog.org

http://www.cdc.gov/ncidod/nip

http://www.fns.usda.gov/fns/

http://www.cdc.gov/

http://www.ask.hrsa.gov/MCH.cfm

http://www.cdc.gov/hiv

http://www.cdc.gov/ncidol/dbmd/gbs

http://www.cdc.gov/ncidod/diseases

http://www.cdc.gov/nchstp/dstd/dstdp.htm

http://www.cdc.gov/ncbddd/fas/fasask.htm

http://www.cdc.gov/ncidod/diseases/hepatitis/index.htm